T0144667

THE HEALTH BENEFITS OF RIBOSE

The All-Natural Energy Booster

PAUL ADDIS, Ph.D.

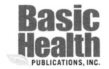

Basic Health
PUBLICATIONS, INC.

The information contained in this book is based upon the research and personal and professional experiences of the author. It is not intended as a substitute for consulting with your physician or other healthcare provider. Any attempt to diagnose and treat an illness should be done under the direction of a healthcare professional.

The publisher does not advocate the use of any particular healthcare protocol but believes the information in this book should be available to the public. The publisher and author are not responsible for any adverse effects or consequences resulting from the use of the suggestions, preparations, or procedures discussed in this book. Should the reader have any questions concerning the appropriateness of any procedures or preparation mentioned, the author and the publisher strongly suggest consulting a professional healthcare advisor.

Basic Health Publications, Inc.
www.basichealthpub.com

ISBN: 978-1-59120-170-0 (Pbk.)
ISBN: 978-1-68162-809-7 (Hardcover)

Copyright © 2007 by Paul Addis, Ph.D.

All rights reserved. No part of this publication may be reproduced, stored in a retrieval system, or transmitted, in any form or by any means, electronic, mechanical, photocopying, recording, or otherwise, without the prior written consent of the copyright owner.

Editor: Roberta W. Waddell
Typesetting/Book design: Gary A. Rosenberg
Cover design: Mike Stromberg

Contents

*To Evie, my wife of thirty-nine years,
and the sweetest person I know.*

Acknowledgments

Several colleagues devoted significant amounts of time and effort reviewing this book in manuscript form, making useful suggestions and helping with figures, and their help is hereby gratefully acknowledged. Clarence Johnson, Ph.D., and John St. Cyr, M.D., Ph.D., were very helpful with regard to the science of ribose and its benefits for humans. Mike Wright and Jackie Menne performed an excellent service on the figures. Mr. Wally Wilsey, President of Red Oak Management is appreciated for introducing me to the newer findings on ribose and human disease, and for advice on the manuscript. Terry Stewart also had some useful suggestions and his inputs are appreciated. John Foker, M.D., Ph.D., should be recognized because it was his work at the University of Minnesota that really stimulated the exciting findings on ribose that today are responsible for advancing human health in several important fields of medicine. Last but not least, I thank my editor, Roberta W. Waddell, for her tireless efforts to keep me focused on simplifying the complex scientific phenomena discussed in this book so the average non-scientist can understand it.

1. What Is Ribose?

Ribose is a naturally occurring sugar produced in the body from another sugar called glucose (or sometimes dextrose). As such, ribose shares many properties of glucose, and other sugars, such as fructose and galactose. However, ribose is made of only five carbon atoms compared to six carbons for the other three sugars. Six-carbon sugars are burned for energy, but ribose is *not*. There is very little ribose in the diet of man. And, although the body makes ribose from glucose, obtainable in the diet from table sugar and complex carbohydrates, the conversion of glucose into ribose is slow. The body, therefore, tries its best to conserve ribose, keeping it available to fill a critical role in countless functions of cells and tissues.

Life itself depends on a chemical-energy molecule called adenosine triphosphate (ATP). This compound provides all the energy needed to maintain cellular integrity and function, and ribose is the structural backbone of ATP. Ribose is essential for literally thousands of chemical reactions in the body, and is used as a regulator and an energizer for virtually all cell functions. It also provides a pivotal part of deoxyribonucleic acid (DNA), our genetic code, and an information library for the body. A simplified diagram of ATP, showing the ribose framework of the molecule, is presented in Figure 1.1.

WHY THE SUDDEN INTEREST IN RIBOSE?

As a dietary supplement, ribose is receiving greatly increased attention because recent research has shown that it is crucial to many health issues, and that it is generally in short supply in the body. Ribose is

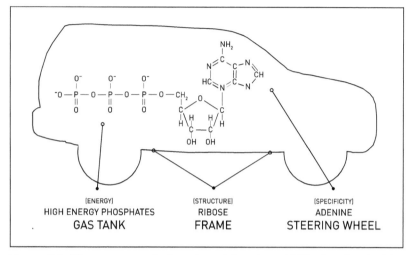

Figure 1.1. The structure of adenosine triphosphate (ATP), the chemical (or usable) form of energy needed by cells and tissues has been superimposed over a graphic of an automobile for purposes of illustration. Ribose plays a crucial role as the central structural element of ATP, connecting adenine, the steering wheel that guides ATP to the proper place in the cell, to the triphosphate group, the gas tank. The energy is stored in the chemical bonds that hold the phosphate groups together. These are called high-energy phosphate bonds.

extremely beneficial in treating or preventing three very consequential diseases: Chronic fatigue syndrome, fibromyalgia, and heart problems, including congestive heart failure and ischemic heart disease. Ribose assists the body in maintaining a normal blood-sugar level (it is a useful tool in treating diabetes), and in controlling appetite and weight gain. Supplementing with ribose has been shown to augment your exercise program, in itself an important health-enhancer. Even bodybuilders and weightlifters find that ribose is supportive in their attempts to build great bodies. But perhaps the most remarkable benefit of ribose supplementation, one you can notice almost immediately, is the protection it gives your muscles when you push yourself too far in physical work. Your muscles will be protected from fatigue and, more important, from soreness caused by muscle exhaustion.

The roles of ribose in many other health-related areas are being actively studied at this time. One exciting area is that of brain metabolism and neurological disorders, such as Alzheimer's and Parkinson's disease. In terms of its energy metabolism, the brain has many features in common with the heart and muscle. It has been hypothesized that ribose could boost the energy of brain tissue. This could be significant because it has been shown that in Alzheimer's and Parkinson's diseases, ATP levels are low and the reduced levels play a role in these and other neurological disorders.

Ribose possesses unique properties that enable it to trap building blocks of energy in cardiac (heart) and muscle cells, allowing for an improved recovery after a heart attack, a better avoidance of the incapacitating nature of congestive heart failure, an improvement in the conditions associated with fibromyalgia, and recovery from exhaustive physical exercise.

Another reason for the sudden interest in ribose is that the stressful lives many people now live deplete ribose in the body and it can't be replaced fast enough, hence a need to supplement. Taking ribose will help you have more energy to work longer and better, think more clearly, and feel less pressured or depressed. All these benefits explain the rapidly increasing use of ribose, now found in more than seventy-five products. One teaspoon of ribose powder mixed into a glass of fruit juice is a typical dosage for better health maintenance.

RIBOSE—A SCARCE COMMODITY

There are no good natural sources of ribose in your diet and, until recently, there have been no good sources for supplemental ribose.

A simple fermentation is now used to convert glucose to ribose in a process that imitates the body. The body *does* make ribose from glucose but does so very slowly. Its production in the body appears sufficient for its normal needs in daily activities, but in today's stressful times, including diseases and exercise, the body cannot make ribose fast enough. Ribose supplementation is not necessary for life, but it certainly enhances your health and wellness.

Ribose is an advantageous nutritional supplement for several reasons. It is a vital component of every cell, and life itself depends upon ribose. As a supplement, ribose is entirely safe, because it is an exact replica of the substance produced by the body. Also, the body recognizes the crucial role of ribose. The body does not burn it as fuel, but rather conserves it for other crucial physiological roles. Further, ribose supplementation is effective at relatively low levels, another margin of safety. There are no contraindications to supplementing with ribose. Taking ribose does not cause a spike in blood sugar so it is safe for people with diabetes, although people with type 1 diabetes who are taking ribose need to test their blood sugar to make sure it does not go too low. No difference exists between a person with diabetes and someone without, in terms of ribose metabolism, and if anything, supplemental ribose in the diet of a person with diabetes appears to aid in the control of sugar. There are no other chemicals, pharmaceutical drugs, or supplements that can substitute for ribose. Since the body does not store ribose efficiently, it is most effective taken as a daily supplement. A teaspoonful of the powder in your orange juice or on your cereal is all that is required, although larger doses may be suggested by a nutritionally-aware doctor for congestive heart failure, fibromyalgia, heart disease, or other conditions that may require continual energy enhancement.

WHAT ARE SOME STRESS CONDITIONS THAT REQUIRE RIBOSE?

In connection with the body, the word stress is used broadly as any condition that interferes with the production of energy in cells, or any condition where supply does not meet demand. This could be something as simple as exercise, or as profound as coronary heart disease or congestive heart failure. In this book, I will elaborate on the number of diseases and conditions for which ribose can be helpful, in the process giving you an understanding of how food is burned and converted to ATP energy. The narrative of the importance of ribose to your health is not only crucial, but also extremely interesting. It is a fascinating journey.

IS RIBOSE AN ESSENTIAL NUTRIENT?

Ribose, glucose, and other sugars that belong in the carbohydrate class are absolutely necessary for life and are therefore nutrients. Yet, since the body makes them, they might not be considered *essential* nutrients, those nutrients that must be provided by the diet to support life. The fact is, ribose is essential for life to exist and although the body *can* produce enough to support life, neither the body nor the typical diet supplies enough ribose to provide for recovery from stress, or ensure an *optimal* life. So from this point of view, ribose could be considered an essential nutrient.

WHY YOU SHOULD READ THIS BOOK

This book will discuss how your body works and the biochemistry of life itself, with particular reference to ribose and its benefits. It details the importance of ribose in treating cardiovascular problems and fibromyalgia, and shows how ribose may help keep you healthy by enhancing your exercise program, thereby reducing your susceptibility to cancer, diabetes, heart disease, hypertension, obesity, and strokes.

WHY YOU CAN RELY ON THE INFORMATION IN THIS BOOK

Hundreds of books on supplements, diets, and weight loss have been written, but most of them rely solely on anecdotal information. In the weight-loss field, diet books have been produced for more than fifty years, with most promoting an unhealthy diet, and only a few based on scientific data published in peer-reviewed medical and scientific journals. Proof of the failure of these anecdotal weight-loss books is the unavoidable fact that obesity is a bigger problem today than at any time in America's history.

The book you are about to read is vastly different in two respects. First, all information presented is based on soundly researched scientific studies published in peer-reviewed scientific journals. If, for example, ribose is said to be beneficial in treating congestive heart failure, this statement is based on more than a hundred scientific publications. Second, you will be given enough scientific background to have a good, practical understanding of how ribose works in your body. This will enable you to make a sound scientific decision regarding whether or not you want to supplement with ribose. Also, your insight into the biochemistry of ribose will help you avoid unhealthy treatments or diets.

2. Metabolism—Converting Food into Energy and Using It

The most critical aspect of metabolism involves burning carbohydrates, fats, and proteins to produce carbon dioxide, water, and energy. The energy is trapped in the adenosine triphosphate (ATP) molecule, the chemical form of energy and the most vital chemical in the body. Ribose provides the structural backbone of ATP.

Before discussing how food energy is converted into chemical energy and how the body uses chemical energy, it is important to appreciate just how important ATP really is to living tissue. Everyone is familiar with the term *brain dead,* and the reason invariably given for this situation is lack of oxygen. But is it really lack of oxygen? In reality, the death of any tissue is not due to lack of oxygen, but rather to lack of energy. The tissue simply runs out of ATP. As strange as it may sound, the fact is that many living organisms flourish without oxygen (they are anaerobic), and some, such as botulism bacteria, cannot even tolerate it, but life cannot exist without ATP.

Oxygen is important in aerobic organisms, of course, because much of the ATP produced comes from metabolism that uses oxygen. But it is the loss of ATP that ultimately leads to the death of cells, tissues, and eventually the entire organism. This is the reason why ribose is so important—it makes ATP and keeps ATP levels high enough to sustain life.

Many common conditions can result in a loss of ATP, and low ATP levels, if severe enough, can make it almost impossible to manufacture new ATP. This is where ribose comes in. If there is a crisis, such as a heart attack, providing extra ribose can help to recharge life-sustaining ATP.

When you ingest food, it is digested into smaller units, absorbed into the blood, and placed into the appropriate cells, where metabolism begins. Metabolism can be a difficult subject to grasp, but the effort is well worthwhile, and the subject is extremely interesting. The story of how life itself is maintained is basically the story of metabolism, and learning about cellular metabolism will give you the tools you need to understand many other related areas of great importance to your health. In this complex story of ribose and metabolism, I use illustrations and analogies to make the subject comprehensible, applicable, and just plain fun.

A BRIEF OVERVIEW OF METABOLISM

Metabolism is defined as the total sum of all the chemical processes occurring in the body. These reactions enable cells to release energy from food and use the generated energy to perform muscular work and other tasks within the cell. There are two sides to metabolism. Catabolism is the breaking down of large molecules into smaller ones, ending with carbon dioxide, water, and the production of energy in the form of ATP. The other side of metabolism is anabolism, the use of ATP to make large molecules, such as proteins and other cellular components, perform work and do other vital tasks within the cell.

Glycogen, also called animal starch, provides a fine example of ATP production, including the concepts of anabolism and catabolism. Glycogen is a large structure comprised of up to 400 glucose units bound together. Glycogen serves as one of the primary potential energy sources for muscles. To produce energy from glycogen, muscle cells break it down into its component glucose molecules (catabolism), each of which contains six carbon atoms. Catabolism continues as glucose is further broken down to six carbon dioxide (CO_2) molecules and six water molecules ($6H_2O$). This phase of catabolism uses oxygen and produces a large amount of ATP.

Anabolism is best illustrated by the synthesis of proteins. A good analogy for this is to visualize railroad freight cars being hooked together by a switch engine, which uses energy to push the cars with enough force to couple them and make them into a whole long freight train. Protein production begins with at least two amino acids joining together. ATP is required for this reaction. Then a third amino acid is added to the other two, and another ATP molecule is used. This process continues until a long protein (train) is completed and many ATPs have been used. Ribonucleic acid (RNA) and deoxyribonucleic acid (DNA), containing ribose and deoxyribose respectively, are the directors of protein synthesis in the cells.

After a strenuous contest, an athlete usually experiences some muscle damage and loss of muscle protein. Ribose helps to reverse this loss of muscle protein by aiding the resynthesis of ATP, supplying the building blocks of RNA needed to direct the process, and powering the synthesis of new replacement protein (anabolism).

HOW ENERGY IS OBTAINED FROM CARBOHYDRATES AND FATS

Catabolism occurs largely in metabolic pathways, a series of chemical reactions that, step by step, transform molecules until all the energy has been extracted. These metabolic pathways are somewhat similar to traveling down interstate highways. For example, while your car may look the same as you drive it down the interstate, it is using gas and lowering its energy content. Similarly, in a catabolic pathway, energy is extracted from a compound as it passes down the metabolic highway.

Figure 2.1 on page 9 outlines the main pathways in catabolism, the breaking down of food chemicals for ATP energy production. About fifty chemical reactions have been condensed into a simple diagram. Each reaction usually requires one or more cofactors (coenzymes or minerals, such as calcium, magnesium, or other chemicals). Not every reaction pro - duces ATP. Sometimes several steps are required for one ATP molecule to be produced. The ATP production pathways are carefully controlled by such factors in the body as hormones, nerves, and nutritional status, but its production is strictly dependent on the availability of ribose.

CATABOLISM OF CARBOHYDRATES

The catabolism of carbohydrates occurs in three phases: Phase I, glycolysis; Phase II, the citric acid cycle (CAC) or Krebs cycle; and Phase III, the electron transport system (ETS). Each of these will be discussed in relation to how they supply energy to the cell, and how ribose fits into

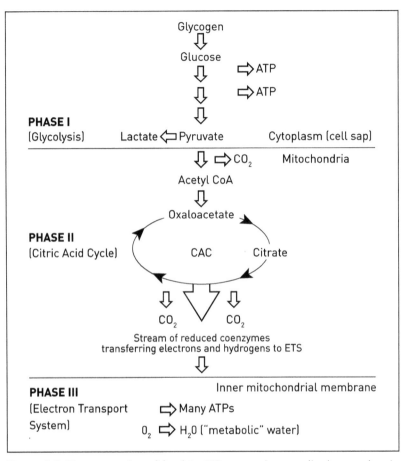

Figure 2.1. The conversion of food to ATP energy is exceedingly complex. In this figure, a metabolic highway of carbohydrate catabolism to ATP is presented in a highly simplified format. (Fats and proteins may also be catabolized to ATP but these metabolic highways are not shown.) The scheme is divided into three phases. In Phase I, called glycolysis, glycogen and glucose are catabolized to pyruvate or, if oxygen is not present, to lactate. In two steps, ATP is manufactured from the energy taken from the molecules in the glycolysis pathway. In Phase II, called the citric acid (CAC) or Krebs cycle, pyruvate enters the mitochondrion by giving up a carbon dioxide (CO_2) molecule. Two additional CO_2 molecules are lost in the CAC. Hydrogen atoms (hydrogen ions plus electrons) are extracted from the many compounds in the CAC and these enter Phase III, called the electron transport system (ETS). In this amazing process, oxygen is used to accept the hydrogens and electrons and forms water. In this process, many ATPs are produced. The overall process is what is known as *respiration*.

the energy equation. The first part of catabolism is glycolysis (Phase I of Figure 2.1). Glycolysis is the process the cell uses to break down sugar. The process occurs in the cytoplasm of the cell, which is the liquid part of the cell containing all the other cellular constituents. Glycolysis also refers to the breaking down of glycogen, which is the glucose storage form found in the liver and muscles. The glycolysis pathway in muscles can be likened to the Indy 500 Speedway, for it is this pathway, more than any other, that can provide explosive bursts of energy (ATP). It is also an example of living (temporarily) without oxygen because glycolysis can produce ATP whether or not oxygen is available. The only difference between the two types is that aerobic (with oxygen) glycolysis stops at pyruvic acid (that then turns into the CAC pathway), whereas anaerobic (without oxygen) glycolysis stops at a dead-end chemical called lactic acid (lactate). Although it can produce explosive bursts of energy, glycolysis can only produce a small amount of ATP, whether oxygen is available or not. In muscle tissue, where energy demands are great, only about 1 percent of the muscle weight is glycogen. Using this glycogen for energy production would allow you to run a fast race but not a long one.

Many metabolic pathways may generate energy from the intermediate chemicals in that pathway, and so it is with glycolysis. In glycolysis, two ATP molecules are harvested (see Figure 2.1) and there is no need for oxygen in these two ATP-producing reactions. Therefore, in an emergency, ATP can be produced very quickly, without having to wait for respiration to feed oxygen into the system. No matter how ATP is manufactured, however, ribose is an essential part of its structure (see Figure 1.1). Normally the ribose used to make ATP does not need to be replaced or supplemented by dietary sources. However, in abnormal circumstances supplemental ribose is a must (these abnormal situations will be discussed in Chapter 6).

ANAEROBIC GLYCOLYSIS

The end-product of anaerobic glycolysis is not pyruvate but rather a closely related chemical called lactic acid, or lactate, which is a toxic by-product of anaerobic glycolysis. Lactate is the acid produced in muscles that is related to the fatigue, soreness, and burning muscles experienced if you exercise too hard. To use the highway metaphor once again, lactic acid represents a dead-end sign in metabolism, and no further metabolism of lactate occurs in skeletal muscle. Instead, the blood removes lactate and transports it to the liver and heart where it can be metabolized by these tissues.

Are you beginning to see the importance of exercise in this picture? People who exercise regularly make extra blood capillaries over time and are therefore able to remove lactate more efficiently during and after exercise. This increases resistance to fatigue, and aids in muscle recovery.

AEROBIC GLYCOLYSIS

The first nine reactions of aerobic glycolysis are the same as in anaerobic glycolysis. However, now oxygen gets involved, and that begins the CAC, Phase II, of the energy process (see Figure 2.1). In aerobic glycolysis, glucose is still converted into two pyruvates. Instead of forming lactate, as in anaerobic glycolysis, these pyruvates take a turn in the highway before reaching the dead end, lactate. This new interstate highway is called the citric acid (CAC) or Krebs cycle, and it leads to Phase III, the electron transport system (ETS). These crucial energy-producing pathways occur in the mitochondria, the tiny powerhouses inside all cells in the body. These mitochondria are the spark plugs of the cell. Think about this as I attempt to explain the CAC and the ETS.

The CAC is named after citric acid, one of its components, which is a principal chemical in citrus fruits. It is also called the Krebs Cycle in honor of its discoverer, Sir Hans Krebs. And he should be honored, as this particular metabolic pathway is *the single most important discovery in the history of biochemistry.*

What is interesting, and in contrast to glycolysis, is that the CAC is truly a cycle, not a pathway. It really is the Indy 500 of the cell, but always operates under a go-slow yellow warning flag. In this pathway, the chemicals go round and round and never really stop. However, if two carbon fragments enter the cycle, something must come out—namely, two carbon dioxides ($2CO_2$). So this really defines the process of respiration—breathing in oxygen (O_2), transporting O_2 to cells, and using it in the process of converting carbohydrates, fats, and even some amino acids to energy (ATP). Carbon dioxide is produced, which is transported to the lungs, and expired back into the environment. All carbon atoms that enter the CAC will eventually be emitted as CO_2.

Many metaphorical references to autos have been used to explain metabolism in humans. One obvious way would be to compare the energy storage and utilization systems of cars and people. They are amazingly similar. Automobile engines use oxygen to burn gasoline, a mixture of chemicals made of hydrogen and carbon (called hydrocarbons) in an internal combustion engine to produce mechanical energy, heat, CO_2, water, and some carbon monoxide (CO). The body's cells also burn chemicals that are various types of hydrocarbons and produce energy in the form of ATP, heat to maintain body temperature, CO_2, and water. The major difference is temperature, with the body running a few hundred degrees cooler than the engine of the automobile. This difference is due to the fact that all the body's metabolic reactions are speeded up and carefully controlled by specialized proteins called enzymes.

As chemicals travel through the CAC, they are steadily degraded in a manner that extracts energy. In fact, by the time CO_2 is formed, virtually all the energy has been extracted. So, from glucose to CO_2, a large amount of energy has been removed. Most of this energy comes from the last part of metabolism, Phase III, the electron transport system (ETS), the most mysterious and miraculous part of metabolism.

There are basically two ways to make ATP. The first, discussed earlier, generates a high-energy structure in the glycolysis pathway. In this pathway, specialized enzymes transfer the high-energy structure from one molecule to the next, making ATP. This process is fast, but not particularly efficient, and will occur with or without oxygen. Not so with the ultimate mechanism of ATP production, the ETS. Here, oxygen is absolutely required, water is produced as a by-product, and a large amount of energy is efficiently produced. ATP is generated from adenosine diphosphate (ADP) and phosphate by removal of hydrogen atoms from the CAC. These hydrogen atoms are then transferred to the ETS in a process that uses oxygen and makes water (H_2O). (See Figure 2.1.) This is often described as a recycling process because of the cyclical nature of the overall reaction. ATP is used by the cell for energy, leaving ADP and a leftover phosphate group (PO_3). The CAC and electron transport chain then put a new phosphate group back onto ADP to re-form ATP. As long as there is enough oxygen supplied to process, this cycle continues unimpeded, billions of times per second in every cell in the body.

The CAC can only operate with oxygen because its main job is to remove hydrogen atoms and transfer them to the ETS. Here oxygen is reduced to water and in the process ATP is produced. Hydrogen atoms are transferred by coenzymes, molecules that are derived from some of the water-soluble vitamins, such as niacin, riboflavin, and thiamin. In the process, one CO_2 molecule is released as pyruvate enters the CAC, and two other CO_2 molecules are released later. The O_2 molecules that are reduced to water in the ETS are what we breathe in, and the CO_2 molecules are what we breathe out in the process of respiration.

Although the CAC produces energy at a slower rate than a really hyped-up glycolysis pathway, it does produce energy more efficiently. Unlike glycolysis, the CAC can also handle fats, which contain nine calories per gram of energy compared to just four calories for proteins and carbohydrates.

Here is a question to ponder that will perhaps help you understand the application of this information. A pheasant is a speedy, explosive, non-migratory bird, and a goose is a migratory bird that flies very long distances. Which of the two kinds of metabolic pathways, glycolysis or the CAC/ETS, would be the predominant one in the flight muscles of each bird? (See Chapter 3 for the answer.)

There are numerous steps in the ETS, and ATP is formed at three specific sites. The overall view of the process of oxidation of pyruvate is that, as it is degraded, hydrogen ions and electrons (hydrogen atoms) are removed and transported to the ETS. Here they pass through six steps. The hydrogens and electrons meet oxygen and form water by a reduction of the oxygen (this is where we can make most of our own water). As this process occurs, ADP plus inorganic phosphate are simultaneously producing ATP.

More than any other life process, the ETS is the basis of life itself in all mammals, and it deserves attention and respect. The ETS also illustrates the crucial role of ribose in the life-giving biochemical mechanism. ATP cannot be made unless there are sufficient levels of ribose inside the cells of the body. The crucial importance of this is nicely illustrated by a calculation presented by Albert Lehninger of Johns Hopkins University School of Medicine and a pioneer researcher of the ETS. He writes, "A normal 68-kg (150-lb) adult requires a caloric intake of 2,000 kcal of food per twenty-four-hour period. This food is metabolized and the free energy used to synthesize ATP, which is then utilized to do the body's daily chemical and mechanical work. Assuming that the efficiency of converting food energy into ATP is 50 percent, calculate the weight of ATP utilized by a human adult in a twenty-four-hour period." The answer is 46 kg (101.2 lb) or 68 percent of the body weight! But the body, at any given time, only holds 50g of ATP, so how can the body make 46 kg (46,000g) of ATP?

Recycling ATP tens of thousands of times a day is the answer to this dilemma. This metabolism can, under certain conditions, result in losses of ATP building blocks from the cells, making it impossible to supply the ATP the body needs. Of course, the cell can employ the pentose phosphate pathway to make more ribose but, as discussed below, it is too slow to be of much help.

THE PENTOSE PHOSPHATE PATHWAY
WHERE RIBOSE IS PRODUCED

The final pathway to be discussed, the pentose phosphate pathway, is where ribose is made. It is interesting, and very significant, that heart and skeletal muscles, the types of tissues asked to do a great deal of physical work and therefore requiring a robust production of ATP, are not enriched with this ribose-generating pathway. In fact, the pentose pathway is not abundant in the tissues requiring the most ATP, and wherever it is abundant, it runs at a slothful rate. For this reason alone, it would behoove people to supplement with ribose for their hard-working muscles or energy-deficient cardiac cells.

The oxidation of glucose is key in this pathway. The product formed by this process is acted upon by another enzyme and eventually a carbon dioxide is removed. As illustrated in Figure 2.2 on the next page, this process converts a six-carbon sugar, glucose, to a five-carbon sugar, ribose.

The brain, heart, and skeletal muscles, which make energy, store energy, and use energy in far greater amounts than all other tissues combined, are the next topics to be covered.

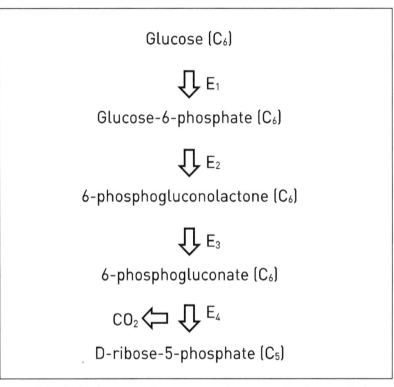

Figure 2.2. The body can use the pentose pathway to make ribose, as is shown above. (Pentose means five-carbon sugar.) The first step converts the hexose, six-carbon sugar, glucose (dextrose) to glucose-6-phosphate. The pentose path - way produces ribose in the usable form of D-ribose-5-phosphate. The two key aspects of this pathway to remember are: first, in tissues requiring lots of ATP, the pentose pathway is ironically slow; and second, in a crisis, the pentose pathway cannot produce ribose fast enough to help maintain critical levels of ATP.

3. How Metabolism Works in Skeletal Muscle, Heart Muscle, and the Brain

Skeletal muscles, those connected to bone, constitute the organ system that is responsible for activity, movement, and work, and they need the greatest amount of energy by far. A second type of muscle tissue is the cardiac muscle that powers the heart. On a pound-for-pound basis, the energy needs and the energy-producing capacity of the heart are simply astonishing (see Chapter 4). A third type are the smooth muscles of the blood vessels and digestive tract, which also use ATP to do work, but in less impressive amounts.

In addition, one other tissue, the brain, requires a surprising amount of energy and its energy metabolism is very similar to that of muscle. With few exceptions, all other tissues, such as the liver, are sluggish with respect to energy metabolism because they do not use ATP to the extent that muscle does.

Large semi trucks that haul big loads for long distances have *two* very large fuel tanks. Similarly, muscle, heart, and even the brain, have storage forms of ATP to help out when necessary.

To comprehend how this system works, it is first necessary to understand how tissues use ATP for various tasks. Assume you are playing softball. If you throw the ball from centerfield to home plate, the reaction that takes place in the triceps muscle of your arm is:

Throwing action* and relaxation:

$$\text{Actin} + \text{Myosin} \longleftrightarrow \text{Actomyosin}$$

Supplying the energy:

$$\text{ATP} \longleftrightarrow \text{ADP} + \text{Pi} + \text{mechanical energy*} + \text{heat}$$

Actin and myosin are large proteins in your skeletal muscle that contract and form actomyosin, a combination of the two proteins. At the cellular level, combining actin and myosin generates the force needed to throw the softball. The reaction forms ADP and inorganic phosphate (Pi), simply meaning that the ATP loses one phosphorus-containing group and becomes ADP and inorganic phosphate. Note that the arrow goes in both directions ($\longleftrightarrow$) because the reaction is reversible. After you throw the ball, your muscles need to relax before the next throw, so the reverse of this reaction represents relaxation in a muscle cell. Researchers B. B. Marsh and J. R. Bendall of Cambridge University in Great Britain figured this out studying whale muscle in the 1950s. They discovered what is now called the relaxing factor of muscle. Believe it or not, there are tiny pumps inside your muscle cells that remove calcium and sort other minerals into their proper places. The work done by these cellular pumps permits the proper control of the contraction (throwing)/relaxation cycle and requires a very large amount of fuel (ATP). This is a vital process in the muscle cell because, if the timely removal of calcium does not occur, calcium will continuously stimulate contraction, setting up an endless utilization of ATP, and causing the death of the muscle cell. In nerves, some believe this phenomenon could possibly be a cause of Alzheimer's or Parkinson's disease.

In the softball-throwing equation, focus briefly on ADP, adenosine *di*phosphate. The energy for throwing the ball came from breaking off one PO_3 (Pi) from ATP. ADP is what remains and it is recycled to again form ATP. There is still energy left in ADP, but when you start breaking ADP down for energy, you are in serious trouble. Using the gas-tank metaphor, you are running on fumes. The ADP breakdown is the first in a series of reactions that eventually leads to the death of muscle and cardiac cells. Boosting ribose levels is the safest way to avoid this cellular death as the unique properties of ribose prevent any leakage of critical building blocks of ATP from the cells (see Chapter 6).

WHY AND HOW HIGH-ENERGY PHOSPHATES ARE STORED IN TISSUE

There are two reasons why certain tissues have elaborate, well-designed methods of storing extra quantities of high-energy phosphates. First and most obvious is, if muscle is asked to do a great deal of work, it just seems like a good idea, the same way it's a good idea to have an extra gas tank for a long trip or highway emergency (see Figure 3.1 below). It is extremely helpful if an emergency occurs—being chased by a black bear

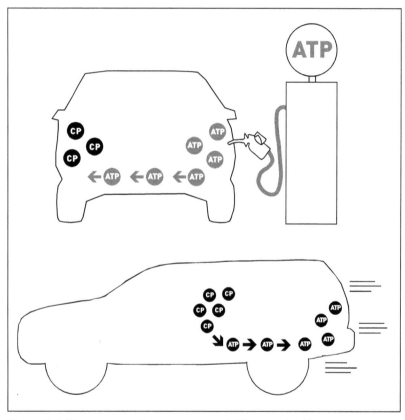

Figure 3.1. The concept of an extra gas tank. The creatine kinase enzyme provides a way to store extra ATP, in the form of an extra gas tank holding creatine phosphate (CP), also a high-energy structure. It can later produce ATP from CP, when ATP levels begin to get significantly lower than at the start of the trip. The first vehicle is shown at a gas station. As tank 1 fills with gas, some is transferred to tank 2, and this continues until both tanks are full—C + ATP ⟶ ADP + CP. The second vehicle is shown moving down the highway, well into its long trip and starting to use some of the gas in the second tank—CP + ADP ⟶ ATP + C. In this example, just as in the human body, the engine must use ATP for energy; it cannot use CP directly, but must first run it through tank 1 (ATP).

or tipping over your boat in the middle of a large lake, for example—to have a readily available source of extra ATP in addition to reserve energy, such as stored fat and glycogen.

Reason number two is more difficult to understand, however. This is the fact that the high-energy phosphate system of storage helps maintain a steady production of ATP. As can be seen in the equation below, the storage of energy in creatine phosphate (CP) also generates ADP, a necessity for the continued production of ATP.

The creatine-kinase (CK) reaction, often called the creatine shuttle, augments readily available fuel stores. As abundant ATP is formed, some is converted to CP, the storage form of ATP. As muscles use the ATP, the reaction reverses and CP supplies energy for the conversion of adenosine diphosphate (ADP) to ATP.

$$\textbf{CK}$$
$$\textbf{ATP + C} \longleftrightarrow \textbf{ADP + CP}$$
$$\textbf{creatine kinase enzyme}$$

adenosine triphosphate $\longleftrightarrow$ **adenosine diphosphate**
creatine **creatine phosphate**

For clarity, let me explain this phenomenon in a different way. To assure that the metabolic pathways, glycolysis and the CAC, can continuously produce ATP, it is necessary for ADP to be available for conversion to ATP. The creatine shuttle helps regenerate ADP by transferring the high-energy phosphate to creatine (to make CP), at the same time making new ADP, which makes good sense for tissues that have large energy demands.

Creatine phosphate is the storage form of high-energy phosphates in cells where energy demands are great. It is the body's second fuel tank, and that is why CK is found in skeletal muscle, cardiac muscle, and the brain.

TYPES OF MUSCLES AND THEIR FUNCTIONS

Have you ever wondered why muscles are so different in terms of coloration? Two examples of big differences are:

- Halibut muscle vs. tuna muscle;

• Chicken leg and thigh muscle vs. chicken breast muscle.

These comparisons reveal some fairly extreme variations in pigmentation that are basically due to the different types of energy metabolism used by each particular muscle, which, in turn, is due to their functions. Before studying skeletal muscle, however, you should appreciate what the heart, a very dark muscle, is able to do as it produces, and uses, an amazing amount of energy. The heart is 25 percent mitochondria by weight (mitochondria are the tiny cellular powerhouses of metabolism—see Chapter 2). To illustrate how fantastic this is, consider that, in some muscles, such as chicken and turkey breast, mitochondria are few and far between, and in many light-colored fish muscles, especially halibut, mitochondria are extremely rare, if present at all.

Muscles can be classified according to their two basic functions, action and posture. Muscles along the vertebrae in the back exemplify the latter type of muscle; they help maintain posture, they are extremely dark, and, similar to the heart, they function almost continuously. As such, these muscles have little need for the explosive energy production of the glycolysis pathway. Instead, for them, the slow, steady CAC/ETS (citric acid cycle/electron transport system) is the prime source of energy.

At the other extreme are the white muscles of birds and some fishes that have tremendous strength, but tire quickly. These white muscles rely primarily on anaerobic glycolysis. The red/white (dark/light) color differences in these muscles are largely caused by differences in the amount of myoglobin they contain. Myoglobin, a colored protein similar to hemoglobin in blood, is the protein that stores oxygen in muscle and heart. This all makes sense because tissues that use glycolysis sparingly, relying mostly on the CAC/ETS, are going to need more oxygen, so it is logical that such muscles need to store more oxygen than halibut muscle, which is almost pure white and contains virtually no mitochondria or myoglobin.

As I said, muscles are either postural or phasic (action-oriented). Postural muscles are dark and act continuously (slowly); phasic muscles can be dark or light, depending on the amount of training these muscles are given. The action muscles can therefore be red or somewhere in between red and white, or almost totally white, giving rise to three types of skeletal muscles.

A fascinating area of muscle biology that will help you understand this important information is the amazing activity of migratory birds. The golden plover, for example, can fly 2,400 miles non-stop across the Atlantic Ocean. These brave birds then promptly leave on the second leg of their journey, covering 2,000 more miles, again crossing the Atlantic, and finally arriving in Argentina.

Stored high-energy phosphates simply will not support this kind of long-distance travel. The amount of ATP that is stored will get the bird flying, and the CP (reserve gas tank) will get it up to speed, but that is about it. The rest of the distance covered must be powered by stored fat, and one characteristic of migratory fowl is their ability to pack away a great deal of fat prior to migration. Another characteristic is the very red flight muscles of their breasts. From this, you can deduce that the bird stores fat and uses the CAC/ETS to produce energy from the mitochondria, burning fat in oxygen delivered by hemoglobin, and stored by myoglobin, while replenishing ATP (and CP) in the process.

Wild ducks and geese also have vividly colored breast muscles and endure a long migration from the Northern tier of the United States and Canada to the Southern gulf states. Prior to embarking, these birds fatten themselves prodigiously and fly daily to engage in muscle training in order to develop the cellular biochemistry needed for their long journey. A notable achievement in birds about to migrate is that they can actually train their muscle cells so that, overall, the muscles become a darker red than before the training period.

In contrast, people who study grouse, pheasant, or quail know that the flight muscles of these explosive, but short-distance flyers, are much lighter in color. Wild turkeys have light gray breast muscles and are amazingly explosive, short-distance flyers. These are huge birds that are muscular and most impressive on takeoff. In human terms, they would be analogous to the body-beautiful weightlifter who would be hard-pressed to run a 10k race. Grouse, pheasants, and wild turkeys are powerful flyers that all use ATP, CP, and glycolysis to power their flight. The fact that they tire quickly proves they have only a modest capacity for the CAC/ETS. (Now you know the answer to the question in Chapter 2 about the type of breast muscle in long-distance vs. short-distance flyers.)

Possessing muscle as white as any, the halibut spends its day lying on the ocean floor, mouth open, waiting for prey to enter. However, if you have ever caught a large halibut, you know firsthand how strong these fish are. But they do tire quickly.

To understand how muscles can differ in coloration, and even more important, how animals, birds, and even people can alter their muscles' capacity for certain types of work through exercise, it is necessary to learn about the different types of muscle cells, how they differ, how they are the same, and how muscle cells are classified into meaningful categories. These categories describe the degree to which each muscle fiber supports either aerobic or anaerobic energy metabolism and also the speed with which each muscle fiber contracts.

CLASSIFICATION OF MUSCLE CELLS INTO THREE FIBER TYPES

Muscles are composed of a varying array of muscle cells, technically called myofibers, or fibers for short. *Myo* is the prefix meaning muscle, and *fiber* describes the fact that most muscle cells (myofibers/fibers) are long and somewhat like a fiber.

After many years of disagreement among muscle biologists on exactly how to classify muscle fibers into a useful system, Dr. C. Robert Ashmore of the University of California, Davis, came up with a simple, brilliant idea. He hypothesized that, with respect to the speed of contraction, there were two fibers, so he designated the Greek letters alpha (α) and beta (β) to denote fast- and slow-contracting fibers (phasic and postural respectively). Ashmore then superimposed either R for red or W for white on these two fiber types. However, it was obvious that β fibers could *not* be white because their tonic activity demanded lots of mitochondria and myoglobin to support it, and that would have made them dark. The α fiber could be expressed as either R or W, depending on the responsibility of the muscle, the activities of the organism, and other factors. Therefore, he called the three fibers βR, αR, and αW.

My colleagues and I demonstrated that this system is consistent with the classification of human muscle fibers. We also showed that, even in the embryonic state, it was possible to differentiate between α and β fibers in several animal species.

TRAINING EXERCISE CAN STRENGTHEN MUSCLES AND IMPROVE FITNESS AND HEALTH

The human body shares a number of characteristics with birds and other animals. Just as migratory birds and mammals can modulate the types of muscle fibers to suit a more aerobic type of metabolism, so can people, if they are willing to get off the couch and start endurance, or training, exercise. The key here is to work intensively enough to require the continuous use of oxygen to burn fat in the CAC/ETS, which requires at least five minutes to activate. The exercise must be intense, last long enough, and be repeated three, four, or five times a week, minimum, to start the ball rolling. To begin with, your αW fibers will, by virtue of their lacking mitochondria and myoglobin, tire quickly. However, as you push yourself repetitively over a period of time, your body will get the message that it can do better. Gradually, most of the muscles you are employing for your exercise program will start making mitochondria, depositing myoglobin, and remodeling αW to αR. Because more mitochondria will require more oxygen to support the oxidation of fats and carbohydrates for ATP production, the muscles will produce new capillaries and therefore improve blood supply. More myoglobin will be synthesized by the fibers for storage of oxygen. As these changes occur, you will notice that it gradually becomes easier to run five miles, swim one mile, or ride a bike 10k. Your body is now much more fit. Your heart also has improved its level of health, as will be discussed in Chapter 4.

HOW DOES RIBOSE FIT INTO THE FITNESS PICTURE?

Migratory birds prove one thing for certain—that endurance types of exercises will burn lots of fat. Birds that complete long migrations have only a small fraction of their original body-fat content when they arrive at their destinations. So, there is much to be learned from these intrepid avian animals. Hard, repetitive exercise requires the production (recycling) of tremendous amounts of ATP and will burn many fat calories.

Stressing-out the muscle may result in losses of ATP, as ADP becomes cannibalized, and the building blocks of ATP are lost from the cell. This problem can only be remedied by taking ribose supplements because ribose traps the ATP building blocks and is essential in synthesizing new ATP to replace that which is lost.

Weightlifters are also well served by ribose supplementation. Although endurance exercise and intensive weight training are quite different in terms of metabolic effects and final results, both types of exercise cause potentially permanent losses of ATP. Heart attacks also causes cardiac muscle cells to resynthesize ATP less efficiently, and this is often permanently true. In all three scenarios, studies have demonstrated there are benefits to be gained by supplementing with ribose.

4. How the Heart Works

The heart is the most important of all the organs in the body and, even with today's technology, it remains almost irreplaceable. This awesome organ is an extremely sophisticated pump that controls the movement of blood through the circulatory system. Further, both the blood and the circulation are amazing. So, before demonstrating how the heart functions, I will briefly discuss the blood and the vessels of the body.

Cardiovascular disease is the leading cause of death in the Western world—with more than 50 percent of all deaths in developed countries caused by diseases of the heart, arteries, and veins. In light of this, understanding the heart, blood, and vasculature (blood vessels) will be very helpful in comprehending the pivotal role played by ATP, and the critical importance of ribose in the overall health of the heart. Over the past two decades, many research studies have conclusively demonstrated the crucial role of ribose in fortifying ATP levels in the heart.

LIFELINES—THE CIRCULATORY SYSTEM

The circulatory system consists of three parts: Blood, heart, and vessels. Each plays its part, and when integrated into one operating system, it is astonishing how it works so well for so long in so many people, despite the abuse heaped on it by poor lifestyle decisions. The blood vessels, or vasculature, consist of a system of continuously branching arteries and capillaries, and a continuously *debranching* system of veins. Arteries transport blood to tissues, and veins remove waste products from cells and tissues and bring them back for processing (removing lactate from tired muscles is an example of this). The waste products are eventually transported to the liver for further metabolism, and CO_2 is shuttled to the lungs for elimination from the body. The really important action occurs at the level of the tiny capillaries, only one cell thick, where the exchange between tissue and blood takes place. The capillary network penetrates into every tissue in the entire body.

Counting the distances covered by all major arteries, smaller arteries (arterioles), capillaries, major veins, and venules, the human body has a circulatory system about 50,000 miles long. Flowing through this inter-state highway of circulation is blood, a remarkable tissue in its own right. Dr. Lester Sauvage, a cardiovascular doctor at the University of Washington, states it best: "Just imagine having to design something that could carry all the chemicals required by the body (including fats, carbohydrates, proteins, and minerals); transport the respiratory gases (oxygen and carbon dioxide); defend the body against infection; be able to seal defects in the walls of injured blood vessels, and still be in a fluid state."

Blood contains many different types of cells. Depending on the level of oxygen, red blood cells (RBCs, or erythrocytes) are what give blood its red color (oxyhemoglobin) in arteries and its blue color (deoxyhemoglobin) in veins. Oxygen is released into the tissues from the blood and it is replaced by carbon dioxide for removal. One teaspoon of blood holds 25 billion red blood cells, and the average person has about 30 trillion of these little cells circulating at any given time. Each red blood cell lives about four months, and then is discarded. Therefore, about one million red blood cells are used up or wear out every two seconds. It is the job of specialized cells in bones to make new RBCs, and this process uses a large quantity of ribose-containing ATP.

Blood also contains (among other things) two additional types of cells: the white cells that fight disease, and the platelets that help blood clot to prevent excessive bleeding. Recent research has shown, however, that both types are involved in the processes leading to heart disease (see Chapter 5).

CHAMBERS, CARDIAC CYCLES, AND CONTROL OF THE HEART

The heart is a marvelously well-designed pump. It has four chambers—two, called atria, are receiving chambers, and two, called ventricles, are for pumping out blood. Although all four chambers have pumping ability, the ventricles are the most powerful in that regard. The right atrium receives the blue-colored, deoxygenated blood returning from various tissues in the body. The right ventricle in the lower part of the right side pumps this blue blood to the lungs where there is an exchange of gasses with the environment. Freshly oxygenated, bright red blood then heads back to the heart, to the left atrium. The left atrium then pumps blood down to the left ventricle, followed by a large push (muscle contraction) by the left ventricle as it pumps blood through the aorta into the arterial system of arteries, arterioles, and microscopically tiny capillaries that feed the tissues.

The average adult heart rate is about 80 beats per minute, as measured by the pulse rate. Do the math. Eighty beats per minute equates to 4,800 beats per hour, 115,000 beats per day, and forty million beats per year. Is it any wonder the heart can show some wear and tear? One way to reduce the total beats per year is to become physically fit (see Chapter 3). An adult in outstanding physical condition will experience perhaps only 50–55 beats per minute at rest. Thirty fewer beats per minute equates to 1,800 fewer beats per hour, 43,200 fewer beats per day, and 15,786,000 fewer beats per year. It makes you want to start an exercise program, doesn't it?

Exercising to strengthen the heart is analogous to what occurs when skeletal muscle is exercised. More capillaries are developed, and the oxygen-requiring ATP-producing system (CAC/ETA) is enhanced. An exercise program can literally help the heart do what it does better than any other organ—repair itself. In order to maintain this system of continual repair, a steady stream of blood must feed the heart muscle itself. This is a different circulatory system than was discussed earlier; this time it is the *coronary arteries,* the part of the circulatory system that is devoted *only* to nourishing the heart. This is crucial to the body because, more than all the other tissues in the body, the heart and the brain depend on a steady supply of blood. If this blood supply is interrupted, even temporarily, death can follow without warning, like a bolt of lightning out of a clear blue sky. A lack of oxygen and low ATP are factors that, occurring together, leave the heart helpless.

Cardiac fibers (muscle cells or myofibers of the heart) have the ability to contract and relax, similar to how skeletal muscle fibers cycle between contraction and relaxation during periods of muscle activity. Pity the poor heart. It never rests. The cardiac cycles occur continuously and must be fully coordinated if the four-chambered pump is to work properly. The cardiac cycle is coordinated by a series of systolic (contracting) and diastolic (relaxing) functions—a system of valves working in concert at a level that would make the Chicago Symphony proud—and an electrical wiring system that makes home wiring look simple by comparison.

Contraction of the heart, called systole, produces a spike in blood pressure as the heart sends blood out into circulation with a fairly strong force. Relaxation of the heart, or diastole, produces a drop in blood pressure. Whenever blood pressure is taken, both numbers are measured and it is this contraction/relaxation cycle that produces the familiar 120/80, systolic over diastolic, blood pressure. These figures are used as one important gauge of the risk for heart disease. Exercise and weight loss are very effective in lowering these values.

Because all four chambers of the heart have a synchronized pumping function, a lack of coordination is disastrous. To avoid this, there are two major coordinating systems—the valves and the electrical system. The valves open and close in an orchestrated manner in order to prevent blood from moving backward in the wrong direction, and to provide a strong surge of blood from the left ventricle into the aorta and the body. The electrical control of the cardiac cycle, systole to diastole, is remarkable. A simplified drawing of the circulatory system is presented in Figure 4.1.

Cardiac fibers are unusual because they can contract on their own in the absence of any activation outside the heart, but if the cardiac pump is going to work efficiently, it is absolutely necessary for it to have a coordinator. To coordinate the heartbeat, there are four specialized nervous systems embedded in the wall of the heart, which conduct waves of electrical impulses. In order, the atria contract first, closely followed by the ventricles: the sinoatrial (SA) node starts the cycle going, and the impulse spreads in all directions through the atria, then moves to the atrioventricular (AV) node, then to the bundle of HIS, and finally to a fourth system, the Purkinje fibers (nerves) that cause the contraction of the ventricles. The reason most cardiac pacemakers are installed is to take over the functioning of this electrical system if it malfunctions.

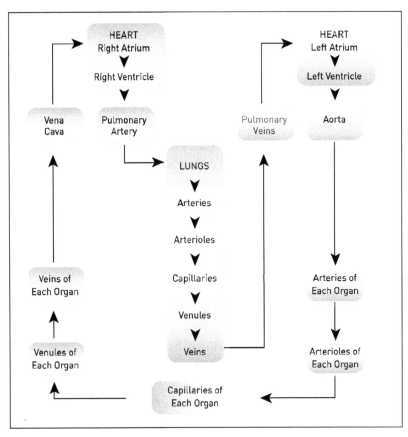

Figure 4.1. A highly simplified diagram of the heart and blood vessels. The exchange of gasses O_2 and CO_2, and the delivery of nutrients to cells and removal of toxins from cells, occurs in the capillaries.

Adapted from Thibodeau, GA. *Structure and Function of the Body.*

SYSTOLIC AND DIASTOLIC FUNCTIONS

The health of both the systolic and diastolic functions in the heart are important. Systole, the contraction of the heart, requires sufficient strength to pump blood into at least 25,000 miles of arteries, arterioles, and capillaries, one-half the total blood-vessel mileage of the human body. Systole also helps the blood make its return trip to the heart, assisted by the veins and venules and covering another 25,000 miles of travel. Pushing billions of red and white blood cells, as well as platelets, through those countless capillaries is no easy task, especially considering that some of the cells, such as the red blood cells, are actually larger than the capillaries they are moving through. If exercise is added to the picture, the heart must respond by increasing the ejection volume and frequency of contractions (heart rate) so the blood flow through skeletal muscle can increase to at least ten times the resting level. This, in turn, requires the heart to substantially increase the recycling of ATP.

In the contraction/relaxation cycle, relaxation is just as important as contraction because, if the heart cannot relax, it cannot fill effectively for the next heartbeat. Relaxation is not a passive process, but is rather an active ATP-requiring process that further adds to the heart's already significant burden of ATP production. In fact, more energy is used in relaxation than in contraction because of the ATP used to seize calcium and pump it out of the cell to permit relaxation. The high-energy requirement of relaxation (diastole) explains the observation that ribose supplementation has its greatest effect when it comes to improving diastolic heart function.

If you consider that the heart may beat 180 times per minute in a young person who is strenuously exercising, the contraction/relaxation cycle is a remarkable process. Now consider that careful measurement of ATP in cardiac cells has indicated that ATP levels provide only enough energy for 10 beats. Add in the creatine phosphate (CP), present at twice the level of ATP in heart muscle, and there is enough for 30 beats or, for the young athlete, about 10 seconds, so it becomes clear that a continual production of energy is essential.

Muscle activity is only one of many ATP uses. Enzymes that break down ATP to ADP + energy are called ATPases. Several are shown in Figure 4.2, illustrating the tremendous burden to produce ATP in cardiac cells. This need to generate energy is where the mitochondria, the powerhouses of the cells, come in, which once again raises the issue of ribose. It is now considered possible that supplementing with ribose will help solve the energy problem and make the system run more smoothly, especially during exercise or a metabolic crisis, such as a heart attack (see Chapter 6 for a detailed discussion of this).

In Chapter 3, I discussed what happens when cellular ATP levels

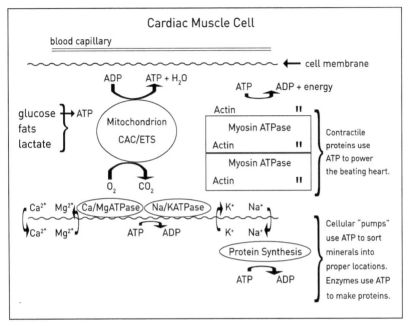

Figure 4.2. This figure illustrates some of the salient features of metabolism in the heart muscle, showing both the production and utilization of ATP and the critical role of ribose in this vital process.

1. ATP production (upper left side of diagram). ATP is produced by burning fatty acids, glucose, and lactate derived from working skeletal muscle in the CAC and ETS located in the mitochondria of the cell. In the CAC, CO_2 is produced and hydrogens and electrons are harvested and enter the ETS. In the ETS, oxygen combines with hydrogen ions and electrons to form water. If a continual supply of oxygen is available to the cell, this process functions normally and produces all the ATP the cell needs to function normally.

2. ATP utilization (right side of diagram). The heart uses ATP in several ways. The most obvious is muscle contraction resulting in the beat of the heart, systole. The contractile proteins, actin and myosin, possess ATPase activity. These ATPase enzymes use the energy supplied by ATP to drive contraction. Adenosine diphosphate and inorganic phosphate are by-products of this reaction. Less well appreciated, but equally critical, uses of ATP are the pumps that shuttle sodium (Na^+), potassium (K^+), calcium (Ca^{2+}) and magnesium (Mg^{2+}) into and out of the cell. These pumps also have ATPases that burn ATP to actually trigger contraction and relaxation (diastole), and they use a large amount of ATP. In addition, all cell components are periodically recycled, replaced, and repaired, entailing a large amount of protein and purine synthesis. These reactions also cause a huge drain on the supply of ATP.

become low. In an effort to make more ATP, the cell cannibalizes ADP: $2ADP \longrightarrow ATP + AMP$. This temporarily solves the low-energy problem, but creates another predicament. The dilemma is that the cell must maintain a specific, constant proportion among ATP, ADP, and AMP to remain healthy. But when the $2ADP \longrightarrow ATP + AMP$ reaction commences, AMP levels change dramatically from very low to very high. This upsets the balance among ATP, ADP, and AMP, and the cellular response is to catabolize AMP to re-establish the proper proportion. But, while lowering AMP levels solves the proportion problem, it creates other, equally serious problems. For example, breaking down AMP into its components allows some of these energy building blocks, called purines, to escape through the cell membrane into the bloodstream, decreasing the total potential amount of energy in the cell. The problem is further complicated by the fact that manufacturing new purines in the muscle and cardiac cell is an extremely slow process. A much better approach, and one that leads to energy conservation, is to trap the purines in the cell. This enables the cell to quickly recover energy levels by re-forming ATP from these components.

This is where ribose comes in. Ribose has unique properties that help to trap purines, preventing their escape from the cell. Supplementing with ribose will increase its levels in the cells, improving the efficiency of the purine-trapping system. If it's available in the cells, ribose will not only retain purines but will help them make ATP quickly.

MITOCHONDRIA IN HEART CELLS

One of the most fascinating aspects of cardiac ATP metabolism is how constant the energy levels remain during rest, light exercise, or heavy exercise, clearly demonstrating that the heart is designed to maintain cardiac muscle-cell viability at all costs. Also, as discussed in Chapter 3, cells do not store large quantities of ATP. The creatine kinase system does store some ATP, as CP, but even CP is not present in large quantities. So, with only limited quantities of ATP and CP in the gas tank, the heart solves the problem of needing huge amounts of energy by packing in large numbers of mitochondria—an astounding 25 percent of the mass of the heart is mitochondria, which gives the heart the ability to recycle ATP very quickly, as long as oxygen is available. Although ATP +

CP levels in cardiac cells will only support about 30 heartbeats, the heart recycles ATP very rapidly, so it is able to continually power the contractions of the heart muscle, synthesize proteins, maintain chemical potentials, and pump calcium.

At Harvard University Medical School, Dr. Joanne Ingwall's experiments and calculations led her to conclude that the heart holds less than one gram (about 0.7) of ATP, but produces 6,000 grams of ATP each day in its energy recycling processes. This is an incredible quantity. Think of it, 6,000 grams equals about thirteen pounds of ATP, or ten times the weight of the entire heart. These resting values are even more impressive in exercising adults. Studies have shown that heart-energy output is carefully matched to the demand. It increases during exercise and slows at rest.

Dr. Ingwall also stated that the heart is omnivorous in that it can convert the energy of an impressive array of carbon-based nutrients into ATP. The mitochondria of heart cells gobble up fatty acids, glucose, ketones, lactate, and pyruvate. The fact that the heart is an omnivore with respect to energy nutrients may be considered its adaptation to its extreme energy requirements.

Now consider that oxygen must be continuously supplied to the heart to support this huge production of high-energy ATP. For many people, this is no problem because they can increase their breathing rate, and deliver oxygen to the heart to support ATP-synthesis by mitochondria. However, if the oxygen supply to the heart were to be suddenly cut off by a blockage in a coronary artery, the heart could no longer produce ten pounds of ATP per day by oxidative metabolism. That would be a disaster, commonly known as a heart attack (see Chapter 5).

5. Coronary Heart Disease and Congestive Heart Failure

Chapter 4 discussed what an energy-producing and energy-using phenomenon the heart is, and how critically the heart depends on a constant flow of blood to support its tremendous oxygen demand. This chapter is about what happens if the blood supply is shut off.

HOW TO FIGHT CORONARY HEART DISEASE AND CONGESTIVE HEART FAILURE

There are a few simple rules you can follow to keep your heart and your arteries in good health.

- Stop smoking because smoking kills more people by cardiovascular disease than it does by lung cancer.
- Eat reasonably. You do not have to become a vegetarian, but you do need to eat lots of fruits, vegetables, and whole grains, and consume fish with a high content of omega-3 oils at least twice a week.
- Maintain a reasonable body weight and normal blood pressure.
- Strictly limit fried foods.
- Ask your healthcare professional about taking a baby aspirin once a day, or a large aspirin once a week.
- Exercise regularly and reasonably.
- As the old joke goes, choose your parents wisely.

Table 5.1 shows the major causes of death in the United States. As you can see, coronary heart disease (CHD) is the biggest killer. Diabetes and strokes are also significant causes of death. All three of these diseases involve the arterial system, are related to diet, and may well be beneficially affected by ribose supplementation. Ribose comes into play in cardiovascular health because of its important role in supporting ATP restoration and retention in cardiac muscle.

TABLE 5.1. MAJOR CAUSES OF DEATH IN THE UNITED STATES ANNUALLY		
Rank	**Cause of Death**	**Percent of Total**
1	Coronary heart disease*	31
2	Cancer	23
3	Stroke*	7
4	Diseases of lungs	5
5	Pneumonia, influenza	4
6	Accidents, including alcohol	4
7	Diabetes*	3

* Note: Diseases with an asterisk indicate that arteries are either primarily or secondarily involved, as is the case in diabetes. In either case, blood flow to the tissues is restricted, damaging or killing the cells. Not all diseases are listed, and for that reason, the figures do not total 100.

CHD—HOW A HEART ATTACK OCCURS AND WHAT IT DOES TO THE MYOCARDIUM

The traditional view of coronary heart disease (CHD), that cholesterol plops down on the artery, is erroneous and outdated, even counterproductive, because it steered people in the wrong direction and promised more benefits than it delivered. The actual process leading to disease of an artery of the heart, and the possibility of a heart attack, is extremely complex. To understand how a heart attack occurs, it is important to refer to Table 5.2 on page 36 and learn some of the relevant technical terms.

THE THREE MAJOR PHASES OF CORONARY HEART DISEASE

In the early 1980s, I began to study CHD seriously for the first time. Reviewing the vast scientific and clinical literature on the subject was

TABLE 5.2. MEDICAL TERMS FOR CORONARY HEART DISEASE AND HEART ATTACKS	
Medical Term	**Description or Definition**
Angina pectoris	Chest pain associated with arterial blockage in heart.
Arteriosclerosis*	Hardening of arteries during aging.
Atheroma	Technical term for plaque.
Atherosclerosis*	Hardening of the arteries with accompanying accumulation of plaque.
Congestive heart	Damage to the myocardium is extensive enough to reduce pumping capacity of the heart, leading to insufficient oxygenation of tissues, especially muscle.
Ischemia	Lack of blood flow through tissues, including the heart, that reduces or stops oxygen supply and reduces or stops the blood from carrying away toxic metabolic products, such as CO_2 and lactic acid.
Myocardial infarction	Technical term for a heart attack, including damage to the myocardium (heart muscle).
Thrombus	Blood clot, the initiator of most heart attacks.

* Note: Although not strictly correct, the terms atherosclerosis and arteriosclerosis are often used interchangeably.

difficult and confusing, so I tried putting the various phases of CHD in chronological order.

I found there are three main stages of the disease: initiation; atherosclerosis, the process of plaque accumulation and thickening of the artery wall; and the terminal stage, thrombosis, a blood clot blocking the flow of blood to the myocardium.

The surprising part of the information is the tremendous complexity of a disease often explained as being caused by too much cholesterol in the bloodstream. In reality, all manner of blood cells, white cells, platelets, and even red blood cells, are involved. Red blood cells have no direct involvement, but there is evidence that regular blood donations are good for the heart (as well as the soul) because they may reduce the viscosity of the blood, making it more watery and less like honey, and permitting the heart to pump more easily. The core of this disease, however, is the involvement of white cells and platelets.

After the heart disease is initiated by an insult to the endothelial cells that line the inside of the artery, white cells and platelets adhere to the damage and try to repair it. Inflammation is part of the disease process, and inflammation of the endothelium is triggered by the activity of white blood cells. Antioxidants help to retard atherosclerosis by inhibiting the activity of white cells that, in addition to their inflammatory activities, also tend to oxidize LDL (the harmful cholesterol), increasing its atherosclerotic activity.

White cells and platelets fix the damage so the artery stays intact, but in the process, the second stage of CHD—atherosclerosis and the associated thickening of the artery wall—gets started. And, once started, this arterial thickening seems to progress for the life of the individual. Blood platelets are crucial in this thickening phenomenon, which is why, if platelets are kept happy, they won't want to hold a convention at the injury site, and the progress of plaque buildup can be slowed. Low serum cholesterol also helps to slow the accumulation of plaque because plaque is partially composed of cholesterol. As the disease progresses, the lumen, or inside diameter, of the coronary artery eventually becomes smaller and smaller, restricting the flow of blood. It is at the second stage, arterial wall thickening, that the oxygen deprivation of the heart becomes serious enough to cause energy levels in the heart to fall dramatically. Therefore, at this stage, the symptoms of angina pectoris or chest pain during physical activity, rest, or even sleep, become apparent.

The final stage is now set. The orchestra has played the overture. Unfortunately, the opera begins and closes in a period of seconds and, as with many operas, it has a tragic outcome. If professional advice to eat salmon twice a week and maybe take a baby aspirin daily is ignored, a blood clot can form, move down the artery where the lumen is much smaller in diameter due to arterial wall thickening, and severely or totally shut down the blood supply to the heart muscle fed by that artery. (Vitamin E, the most famous of all antioxidants, can also help to inhibit platelets.) The technical term for this is ischemic heart disease and it ends in a myocardial infarction (MI). What it means literally is that a heart attack has occurred because the blood flow has been shut down to a portion of the heart muscle. No oxygen is being delivered to that area of the heart muscle, it has used up its energy supply and has become energy-starved, and the toxic products of *anaerobic* metabolism, such as lactic acid, are accumulating.

Refer back to the earlier discussion of how metabolism is either aerobic, efficiently producing CO_2, H_2O, and ATP as end products in the CAC/ETS, or anaerobic, producing some ATP and much lactate, in the glycolytic pathway. Also, recall that the heart is a genuine aerobic metabolic machine, with one-quarter of its weight in mitochondria.

Lactic acid is one of the most important factors causing fatigue and stiffness in muscles that are strenuously exercised without being properly trained. Imagine what damage may occur in the heart if it is forced to continue to work, but the flow of blood is restricted. What occurs is the accumulation of lactic acid, a lowering of its pH, the destruction of enzymes crucial to metabolism, the damaging of the membrane, and the associated leakage of enzymes and other cell constituents into the bloodstream that would not normally be present in the blood. In this regard, one of the prominent enzymes that leaks out of the cell during a heart attack is creatine kinase. Measuring the creatine kinase level in the blood is the basis for one of the tests used to determine whether or not you have experienced an MI, or simply have indigestion.

What happens to the myocardium during an MI is that some of the cardiac muscle fibers become anoxic and energy-depleted. These muscle cells die, and depending on the total amount of damage, the person may die, experience debilitating effects, or be very lucky. Often the sequel to an MI can be congestive heart failure, another condition related to coronary disease. A congested heart means that the myocardium has basically lost some of its pumping power. As a result, the person feels tired, does not want to exercise, and simply prefers a continuation of the sedentary lifestyle that got him or her in trouble in the first place. But, even worse, unless the individual who has congestive heart failure gets off the couch, the prognosis is poor. The congested heart can become so weak that fluid begins to pool in the legs, and eventually in the lungs and heart itself, a dire situation. A great amount of research has shown that the way to get the person moving again is to provide dietary ribose, which will boost energy levels in both the heart and skeletal muscles and allow them to overcome fatigue and begin an exercise program.

HOW TO MINIMIZE THE DAMAGE AND REGENERATE THE CONGESTED HEART

Should you first call 911, then take an aspirin, or do the reverse? The reverse is the correct answer. Good results have occurred if people chew up and swallow an aspirin at the first sign of an MI, then call 911 and wait for help. *Under no circumstances should you drive yourself to the hospital.* The aspirin will help reduce the size of the blood clot that is forming and blocking blood flow. Another idea is to use ribose regularly. One of the problems the heart has during an MI is keeping the ATP levels high, and ribose can help in this by keeping the building blocks of ATP inside the cell. In the absence of ribose, the components of ATP simply leak out of the cell, never to be seen again. Ribose has such an important role to play, in fact, that it is now being used in a growing number of hospitals to treat people who have already had a myocardial infarction. Finally, if energy levels can be augmented after MI-induced congestive heart failure, you can strengthen your heart, and your skeletal muscles, and the blood flow to each. Ribose helps the congested heart by restoring ATP levels, strengthening the function of the heart, permitting more vigorous exercise programs, and strengthening the overall skeletal and cardiac muscle systems. It also improves the quality of life for people with congestive heart failure.

HOW DIETARY RIBOSE SUPPLEMENTATION CAN HELP FIGHT HEART DISEASE

A heart attack is clearly a life-changing experience. A myocardial infarction is serious, life-threatening, and for too many people, a sudden life-ending event. The lifestyle changes discussed earlier will help, but they will only lower your risk, not eliminate it. Ribose is tantamount to having an extremely effective insurance policy. It allows for a more extensive exercise program to strengthen both heart and skeletal muscles, which stimulates a more aerobic type of metabolism and reduces the risk of a blood clot. However, a heart attack (MI) can occur in anyone at any time, and it is during a heart attack that ribose may have its most crucially beneficial effect. It is well established that an MI severely curtails the oxygen supply to the myocardium and this quickly results in a drastic drop in ATP. It is known that supplementing ribose will boost ribose levels inside the heart cells. Research has shown that ribose prevents some of the building blocks of ATP from leaking out of the cell and helps prevent the drop in cellular energy levels. It is important to remember that, even if the doctor uses clot-busting drugs and opens your blocked artery, if the purine building blocks of ATP are no longer available, plentiful supplies of oxygen will not restore energy. Boosting your ribose levels by supplementing your diet with it may not only help prevent a heart attack, but could help you survive one.

6. How Ribose Helps You Maintain High Levels of Vital ATP

This chapter will provide details on exactly how ribose helps protect and improve the energy levels in skeletal muscles and the heart. It will become clear that ribose can also help those with congestive heart failure or fibromyalgia, and anyone participating in exercise programs or engaging in body strengthening and bodybuilding.

LOSSES OF ATP BUILDING BLOCKS DURING MYOCARDIAL INFARCTION

As noted in Chapter 3, in muscle contraction ATP is broken into ADP + Pi. Normally, the ADP would be sent back to the ETS to be rephosphorylated (re-energized) to ATP. Situations frequently arise, however, that do not represent normal times.

If the oxygen supply to the cell is curtailed, normal energy recycling through the ETS does not function, and cells run out of ATP. There is still one last effort to supply energy to the cell, and that is by gleaning energy from ADP. But the downside is that gleaning energy from ADP is what sets the stage for losses of adenine (and other purines) from the cell that cannot be easily, or quickly, replaced. As Dr. Joanne Ingwall said in her book, *ATP and the Heart,* this loss of energy substrates is "a metabolic disaster." Purines are the chemicals that include adenine, the steering-wheel part of the ATP molecule (see Figure 1.1), and they are vital to cell function.

Pulling the energy out of ADP begins with the reaction catalyzed by the enzyme myokinase (MK), also called adenylate kinase (AK):

$$\text{ADP} + \text{ADP} = 2\text{ADP} \overset{\text{MK}}{\underset{\text{AK}}{\longleftrightarrow}} \text{AMP} + \text{ATP}$$

In this reaction, two ADP molecules are used to produce one ATP, with an adenosine monophosphate (AMP) formed as a second product. The AMP is what causes the problems leading to the loss of hard-to-replace purines. As soon as AMP levels increase, the cell uses not one, but two enzymes to attack AMP and lower its level to re-establish the correct proportion among ATP, ADP and AMP. Also, the cardiac and skeletal muscle cells take forever to make new purines inside the cell. This loss of purines is a metabolic disaster because if the body loses purines, such as adenine, it cannot resynthesize ATP, regardless of how much high-energy potential is produced by the ETS. The earlier discussion describing a heart attack (MI) said that when the doctor re-establishes blood flow, the coronary tissues are once again receiving oxygen, the ETS is transporting electrons, and is ready to trap the energy into the ATP molecule, so we should be set up to make ATP. Unfortunately, if purines have washed out of the cell, the pool of ADP has become smaller and there is not enough ADP left to accept the high-energy bond from the ETS. If the energy supply shrinks, there just isn't enough energy in the cell to drive all the biochemical reactions it needs in order to function normally. The reaction pathway for the heart, associated with this metabolic disaster, is shown below in greatly simplified form.

ATP $\longrightarrow$ ADP $\longrightarrow$ AMP $\longrightarrow$ Adenosine $\longrightarrow$ Adenine

Adenine is a critical purine, and in the absence of the activated form of ribose, called PRPP (see Figure 6.1), the purines simply leak out. All would be fine if the cell could simply take some atoms to use as building blocks and make some new adenine. In the liver, this sequence is fairly fast, but in heart and skeletal muscles, the process takes a long time, and simply will not occur while the tissue is stressed by strenuous exercise or disease. According to Dr. Ingwall, in cardiac muscles it will require at least 100 days under the best of conditions to make the normal level of purines. In someone with a sick or damaged heart, this might as well be forever.

Now, place all this in perspective for a person with chest pains indicating a possible myocardial infarction. These phenomena cannot be overemphasized because they show clearly why supplemental ribose can literally save a person's life. The person with the chest pains chews and swallows aspirin, calls 911, and is rushed to the hospital. At the hospital, all sorts of techniques are used to reopen the artery, including atomic-strength clot-busters to augment the aspirin. Soon, blood flow through the formerly blocked artery begins to bring oxygen to the oxygen-starved tissue. The accumulated lactic acid is carried away, so its toxic activities are curtailed. With fresh oxygen ready and willing to accept hydrogens and electrons to form water in the ETS, energy is ready to be produced. Or is it? To capture the chemical energy ready to be harvested from the ETS, you need to have ADP present in fairly copious quantities because the reaction is:

$$ADP \; + \; Pi \; + \; ETS \; energy \; \longrightarrow \; ATP$$

The key aspect to remember is that, even after the doctor re-establishes blood flow and oxygen supply to the myocardium, a person still may not recover if the purine losses have been severe. In fact, any purine loss is severe. The reason is that ADP is nowhere to be found.

HOW RIBOSE LESSENS LOSSES OF THE PURINES, INCLUDING ADENINE

Ribose undergoes the same digestion, absorption, and assimilation into cells as most nutrients. But once ribose enters cells, it begins its crucial role of helping to synthesize ATP and reduce losses of adenine to aid in the trapping of energy.

This area is very complex. When ribose enters a cell, it is acted on by ribokinase, an enzyme that uses ATP to attach a phosphate to the ribose molecule, creating ribose-5-phosphate. Another enzyme then hits ribose-5-phosphate with ATP to add two more phosphate groups at the other end of the molecule, producing 5-phosphoribosyl-1-pyrophosphate (PRPP), which enters into metabolic pathways that synthesize ATP.

While I was thinking about how best to explain this rather complicated phenomenon in simple terms, two inmates at the local jail were mistakenly released. It then occurred to me, what ribose (actually PRPP) does in the cell is to prevent jailbreaks of purines.

PRPP has unusual and crucial properties that allow it to grab, restrain, or trap, adenine, hypoxanthine, and inosine before they break out of the cell. Since it is crucial to retain purines inside the cell, especially cardiac and skeletal muscle cells that are not very good at purine synthesis, PRPP molecules act as the police, preventing the escape of purines from the cells, keeping the energy substrates intact. In addition to restraining purines from their attempted breakout, PRPP also begins the process of directly making new ATP.

Alert readers may be thinking something just doesn't add up. If it takes two ATPs to convert ribose into the active form, PRPP, why is this so great? Two ATPs to make one PRPP? Where is the energy efficiency in that? The answer is, there *is* efficiency because, once PRPP forms ADP, that ADP can be *recycled*. In fact, ADP gets recycled between ADP and ATP thousands of times an hour, and this is where the fantastic energy efficiency of ribose comes into being.

When hearts and minds are stressed, as they are during high-intensity exercise, or in the case of a heart attack, purines are lost and cellular energy is depleted. This really hurts when the doctor has re-established blood flow in the coronary artery and the mitochondrial ETS is all set to produce ATP, but because of purine losses, has a very limited supply of ADP with which to work. It also hurts physically after strenuous exercise that leaves muscles sore and stiff for several days because they don't have enough energy to recover. Therefore, it seems logical that the two most important properties of ribose, trapping purines and directly aiding in the resynthesis of ATP, can be crucially important both in disease conditions and in healthy tissues that experience metabolic stress. Supplementing the diet with ribose is the one proven method of increasing ribose levels in heart and muscle cells. No drug or other nutrient is able to duplicate the functions of ribose.

In summary, ribose quickly forms PRPP, which acts like the police. Through its action in controlling the salvage pathway, PRPP stops adenine, hypoxanthine, and inosine before they can escape from the cell and, as the driver of ATP synthesis, PRPP accelerates energy recovery. (See Figure 6.1.)

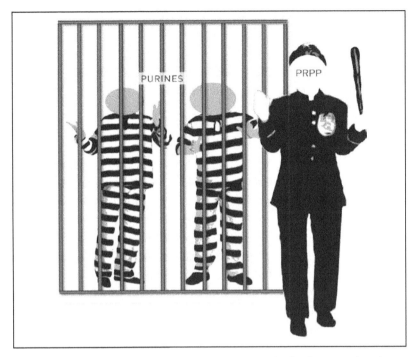

Figure 6.1. This cartoon figure shows ribose, specifically the pyrophosphory-lated form PRPP, acting as the police and preventing the escape of purines from the cell. This permits the cell to use these purine building blocks to resynthesize ATP much faster than having to make purines from scratch and then using them to make the ATP.

In his 2005 book, *The Sinatra Solution: Metabolic Cardiology,* Dr. Stephen T. Sinatra has an impressive list of coronary-health-related issues where ribose can be administered. They are:

- Atrial and ventricular arrhythmia;
- Cardiac diagnosis to unmask hibernating myocardium;
- Congestive heart failure and cardiac hypertrophy, promoting diastolic function;
- Coronary artery disease (coronary heart disease);
- Myocardial preserving agent during cardiac surgery;
- Myocardial preserving agent during PTCA or angiogram;

- Recovery from cardiac surgery or heart attack;

- Stable and unstable angina.

Each of these cardiac issues is highly significant, and all show improvement with ribose supplementation.

RIBOSE, EXERCISE, AND CONGESTIVE HEART FAILURE

It is well established that strenuous exercise can cause muscle changes that are similar to what is happening in the heart during an MI. Lactate accumulates, some damage to muscles and muscle-cell membranes occur, and ADP is broken down to AMP, leading to a loss of purines. Since ribose prevents these losses and speeds the resynthesis of ATP, taking ribose will help a person with a cardiovascular condition begin a more assertive exercise program than would normally be possible, which could help this person achieve a higher degree of physical fitness in a shorter period of time. Another benefit is that it minimizes the fatigue and soreness that often accompanies the commencement of serious exercise in an unfit individual. Improving physical fitness will aid in weight reduction, lower blood pressure, and lower the risk of heart disease. Many people with congestive heart failure have been more than happy to give personal testimonies about how much energy ribose gives them and how much better they feel.

RIBOSE AND WEIGHT TRAINING

Although aerobic (endurance) exercise is the primary recommendation for fighting either coronary heart disease or congestive heart failure, adding some good resistance or weightlifting exercise can also be ex - tremely beneficial. For one thing, as people age, they naturally lose about one pound of lean body tissue (mostly muscle) a year if they do not exercise, and weight training can slow, stop, or even reverse these losses. Secondly, the bones become stronger as muscles are strengthened through weight training. This is important for men, and even more so for women. A third important benefit concerns lean body mass and how it relates to energy use and fat storage. Lean tissue has a higher basal metabolic rate than fat tissue, and weight training can gradually increase

FLOYD'S PROGRESS WITH RIBOSE

Floyd has battled heart disease for many years. At my urging, he tried ribose, adding half a teaspoon to his morning orange juice. He felt better almost immediately, had more energy, did more work around the house according to his wife, Annie, and became more physically fit. After a few weeks on ribose, he decided to stop taking it until he could talk to his doctor, who, unfortunately for Floyd, turned out to be away. These second thoughts caused Floyd to gradually slow down—he felt worse and was much less energetic. To counter this, shortly after the doctor returned from his trip, I provided him with the scientific information on ribose, which allowed him to give the green light for Floyd to resume ribose supplementation. As I expected, Floyd was feeling better very soon. He had more energy, was again helping Annie around the house, and was looking forward to spring and walking, biking, and gardening. Thanks to ribose, Floyd's quality of life—Annie's too—has vastly improved.

the amount of lean tissue, which will, in turn, increase the overall basal metabolism of the body. The importance of this in a weight-loss program is not generally appreciated. It should be, though, because basal metabolism burns, by far, the biggest share of our daily energy needs. The nice thing about basal metabolism is that it burns energy at the same rate whether you are awake or asleep—about one calorie a minute, which amounts to 1,440 calories per day for the average person. The total energy requirement for the human body is only about 1,900 to 2,200 calories per day so it is obvious that any change in basal metabolism is critical. Give it a boost with some weight training.

Another advantage of weight training is that it helps increase resistance to the injuries everyone is susceptible to in everyday life. The sore shoulder or pulled back muscle can be all but eliminated by a sensible exercise program.

I have discussed how daily ribose supplementation enhances an endurance (aerobic) exercise program, but ribose also fits into an anaerobic weight-training program in several ways. First, of course, it supports energy levels in muscle and heart cells—exercise does require ATP. Second, exercise causes some breakdown of muscle protein and, as discussed in Chapter 2, it takes energy (ATP) to make new proteins. Third, ATP is needed to make protein and increase lean body tissues. Since protein synthesis actually takes far more energy than working the muscles in exercise, retaining the purines in skeletal muscle is a critical issue that is successfully addressed by ribose supplementation. Adding ribose supplements to your diet will enhance the energy metabolism of your skeletal muscle much the way they do with heart muscle.

RIBOSE AND FIBROMYALGIA

Among the more recent findings regarding ribose supplementation is its beneficial effect on people who have painful fibromyalgia, with or without the chronic fatigue syndrome that is frequently associated with the disease. These people, for the most part middle-aged women, experience almost constant pain, accompanied by anxiety, depression, headaches, an irritable bowel, muscle stiffness and soreness, overwhelming fatigue, sleep disturbances, and weakness. And unfortunately, most current treatment is not very effective.

The causes of fibromyalgia are not fully known, but are thought to be alterations in brain chemistry, anemia, hormone deficiencies (particularly thyroid), overexertion, parasites, stress, tension, trauma, and viral infections. Muscle biopsies on people with fibromyalgia have shown a number of abnormalities, and many are related, directly or indirectly, to the production of ATP. Individuals with fibromyalgia have lower levels of both ATP and CP, as well as reduced levels of total adenine nucleotides (ATP + ADP + AMP) in their muscles (all three of these adenine nucleotides contain ribose). Also, since ribose quickly becomes PRPP when it enters the cell (this is the cellular policeman that prevents the escape of purines and helps to rebuild stores of ATP), it is believed that oral ribose can help people with fibromyalgia. And, recent studies have confirmed that fibromyalgia symptoms are ameliorated by dietary supplementation with ribose.

Conclusion

There is nothing more important to the viability of a cell than the maintenance of energy (ATP) at high enough levels to be consistent with life. Given the central role of ribose in ATP, and the central role of ATP in life, it is obvious that careful consideration should be given to ribose supplementation. Supplemental ribose is completely safe, an exact replica of the ribose made by the body, and modest amounts of it are effective. Presently, ribose is used effectively for bodybuilding, congestive heart failure, endurance (aerobic) exercise, fibromyalgia, heart disease, and sports activities. And this list is just the beginning. In the future, you can be sure there will be more interesting findings concerning the benefits of supplementing with ribose—another good reason to include ribose in your daily intake of supplements now.

References

Addis, PB. "Classification of skeletal muscle fibers in domestic animals and man." *Malignant Hyperthermia.* (Aldrete, JA, BA Britt, eds.) New York, NY: Grune Stratton, Inc., 1978, 227–232.

Ashmore, CR, PB Addis, L Doerr, et al. "Development of muscle fibers in the complexus muscle of normal and dystrophic chicks." *Journal of Histochemistry and Cytochemistry.* 21:226–278, 1973.

Ashmore, CR, PB Addis, L Doerr. "Development of muscle fibers in the fetal pig." *Journal of Animal Science.* 36:1088–1093, 1973.

Carter, O, D MacCarter, S Mannebach, et al. "D-Ribose improves peak exercise capacity and ventilatory efficiency in heart failure patients." *Journal of The American College of Cardiology.* 45(3 Suppl A):185A, 2005.

Clay, MA, P Stewart-Richardson, D Tasset, et al. "Chronic alcoholic cardiomyopathy: Protection of the isolated ischemic working heart by ribose." *Biochemistry International.* 17(5):791–800, 1988.

Einzig, S, JA St. Cyr, J Schneider, et al. "Myocardial ATP repletion with ribose infusion." *Pediatric Research.* 19:127A, 1985.

Einzig, S, JA St. Cyr, J Schneider, et al. "Maintained myocardial ATP with long term ribose infusion." *Pediatric Research.* 20(4 Pt2):169A, 1986.

Gebhart, B, J Jorgensen. "Benefit of ribose in a patient with fibromyalgia." *Pharmacology.* 24(11):1646–1648, 2004.

Hall, N, PB Addis, M DeLuca. "Mitochondrial creatine kinase: physical and kinetic properties of the purified enzyme from beef heart." *Biochemistry.* 18:1745–1751, 1979.

Harmsen, E, PP de Tombe, JW de Jong, et al. "Enhanced ATP and GTP synthesis from hypoxanthine or inosine after myocardial ischemia." *American Journal of Physiology.* 246(1 Pt2):H37–43, 1984.

Hellsten, Y, L Skadgauge, J Bangsbo. "Effect of ribose supplementation on resynthesis of adenine nucleotides after intense intermittent training in humans." *American Journal of Physiology.* 286(1):R182–R188, 2004.

Illien, S, H Omran, D MacCarter, et al. "Ribose improves myocardial function in congestive heart failure." *Federation of American Societies for Experimental Biology.* 15(5):A1142, 2001.

Ingwall, JS. *ATP and the Heart.* Boston, MA: Kluwer Academic Publishers, 2002.

Lehninger, AL. *Principles of Biochemistry.* New York, NY: Worth Publishers, Inc., 1982.

Omran, H, S Illien, D MacCarter, et al. "Ribose improves myocardial function and quality of life in congestive heart failure patients." *Journal of Molecular and Cellular Cardiology.* 33(6):A173, 2001.

Omran, H, S Illien, D MacCarter, et al. "D-Ribose improves diastolic function and quality of life in congestive heart failure patients: A prospective feasibility study." *European Journal of Heart Failure.* 5:615–619, 2003.

Omran, H, D MacCarter, JA St. Cyr, et al. "D-Ribose aids congestive heart failure patients." *Experiments of Clinical Cardiology.* 9(2):117–118, 2004.

Pauly, D, CJ Pepine. "D-Ribose as a supplement for cardiac energy metabolism." *Journal of Cardiovascular Pharmacological Therapy.* 5(4):249–258, 2000.

Pauly, DF, C Johnson, JA St. Cyr. "The benefits of ribose in cardiovascular disease." *Medical Hypotheses.* 60(2):149–151, 2003.

Pauly, DF, CJ Pepine. "Ischemic heart disease: Metabolic approaches to management." *Clinical Cardiology.* 27(8):439–441, 2004.

Seifert, J, A Subudhi, M-X Fu, et al. "The effect of ribose ingestion on indices of free radical production during hypoxic exercise." *Free Radical Biology and Medicine.* 33(Suppl 1):S269, 2002.

Siess, M, U Delabar, H Siefart. "Cardiac synthesis and degradation of pyridine nucleotides and the level of energy-rich phosphates influenced by various precursors." *Advanced Myocardiology.* 4:287–308, 1983.

Sinatra, ST. *The Sinatra Solution: Metabolic Cardiology.* North Bergen, NJ: Basic Health Publications, Inc., 2005.

Thibodeau, GA. *"Structure and Function of the Body."* St. Louis, MO: Mosby Year Book, 1992.

Index

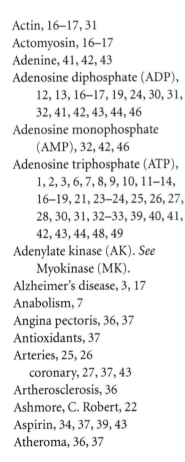

About the Author

Paul B. Addis, Ph.D., is professor emeritus, University of Minnesota, Minneapolis-St. Paul. He received his B. S. at Washington State University and his Ph.D. at Purdue University. He was a Fulbright Scholar in Germany, 1967, and joined the Minnesota faculty in the Department of Food Science and Nutrition that same year. After thirty-seven years, which included thirty-two years teaching the introductory human nutrition course to thousands of students, he retired from the university.

Professor Addis has been published in more than 100 scientific publications and has several patents. His research for these included muscle biochemistry, muscle histochemistry, oxidation of cholesterol in relation to heart disease, and conversion of insoluble fiber from agricultural by-products into soluble fiber, all of which have numerous applications in food processing and human nutrition. During sabbaticals, professor Addis pursued his studies at the University of California/Davis, the University of California/San Diego, and the University of Washington in Seattle. He lives in Cumberland, Wisconsin.

Printed in the USA
CPSIA information can be obtained
at www.ICGtesting.com
JSHW051957150824
68134JS00050B/98